LIZ EARLE'S

Beating
Cellulite

LIZ EARLE'S

Beating Cellulite

BOXTREE

Advice to the Reader

*Before following any advice contained in this book, it is
recommended that you consult your doctor if you suffer from any health
problems or special condition or are in any doubt as to its suitability.*

First published in Great Britain in 1995 as *Liz Earle's Quick Guide
to Beating Cellulite* by Boxtree Limited,
Broadwall House, 21 Broadwall, London SE1 9PL
This edition published in Great Britain in 1996 by Boxtree Limited

The right of Liz Earle to be identified as Author of this Work
has been asserted by her in accordance with the Copyright,
Designs and Patents Act 1988

10 9 8 7 6 5 4 3 2 1

ISBN: 0 7522 0543 9

Text design by Blackjacks
Cover design by Slatter~Anderson

Printed and Bound in Great Britain by Cox & Wyman Ltd,
Reading, Berkshire

A CIP catalogue entry for this book is available from
the British Library

Contents

ACKNOWLEDGEMENTS

I am grateful to Claire Haggard for helping to produce this book. I am also indebted to the talented team at Boxtree, and to Rosemary Sandberg and Claire Bowles Publicity for their unfailing enthusiasm and support.

Introduction

Male doctors and medics may argue that cellulite does not exist, but ask most women and they will confirm that cellulite is indeed a reality. Most of the female population is afflicted with 'orange peel' thighs and dimpled buttocks. It does not make much difference whether you are overweight, as cellulite is just as likely to strike the skinniest bottom. Although not a clinical cause for concern, cellulite does depress those afflicted by it. It is unsightly and can hurt, so what can be done about it? The good news is that there are definite 'cellulite cures' that can help shift the trapped toxins and reduce the build-up of bumpy fat beneath the skin's surface. The bad news is that there is no miracle overnight treatment. It takes time and perseverance to beat cellulite, but with a little help from the right diet, food supplements, body brushing, regular massage and specific exercises it is possible to see a real difference. This book will sort out the facts from the fantasy, and will enable you to make a visible difference to the shape and size of your hips and thighs.

Liz Earle

— 1 —

What is Cellulite?

Cellulite, contrary to the popular view, is a condition with health as well as cosmetic implications. It is said to afflict 80 percent of women in Britain and the USA, in a wide age bracket encompassing puberty and extending beyond the menopause. Despite the numbers of women who suffer from this disfiguring condition, the majority of British doctors remain highly sceptical about the existence of cellulite – in contrast to their European counterparts.

One of the problems is that the subject does not figure as part of conventional medical training, which means that doctors are unwilling to recognise it. Even if privately they cannot deny the existence of cellulite, professionally they are in the dark about what causes it and how to treat it. Out of desperation, many refer their patients for plastic surgery. Progress is not helped by the fact that academics have not exactly been queuing up to undertake research into this particular corner of the dermatological field.

Fact or Fiction?

The issue is further clouded by the fact that cellulite does not fall neatly under the umbrella of either health or illness. Instead, it seems to inhabit the grey area somewhere in between. While it is obviously not a life-threatening condition, the pain, the fluid retention and the localised circulatory problems associated with it are not negligible symptoms. There is also the psychological effect to consider, and the impact of cellulite on some women's lives can be significant. Dr Elizabeth Dancey, who became informed about cellulite treatment when she worked as a GP in Belgium, describes it as a 'benign condition'. She nevertheless concedes that those suffering from cellulite are more at risk from deep vein thrombosis and from infections developing in cellulitic tissue, and she concludes that it is 'not healthy to walk around with kilos of metabolic toxins in your body'.

Cellulite is taken much more seriously on the Continent, and the work carried out by teams of biochemists and dermatological researchers at the Universities of Milan and Toulouse over the past few decades has done much to further our understanding of the condition. 'Cellulite' is in fact a French term, which has been adopted by the international health and beauty fraternity in preference to a clutch of considerably less user-friendly alternatives (imagine trying to squeeze 'localised hydrolipodystrophy' on to a piece of cosmetic packaging!). Not to be confused with 'cellulitis', a medical term which refers to the inflammation of loose connective tissue as a result of infection, cellulite has become the accepted word to describe the 'orange peel' phenomenon which appears on women's hips and thighs.

As yet, there has been no revolution in the British medical establishment's view of cellulite. However, there is at last a flicker of interest in the subject in academic circles. Dr Terence Ryan, consultant dermatologist and clinical professor of dermatology at the Churchill Hospital in Headington, Oxford, far from scoffing at the concept, declares 'mattressing', without hesitation, to be a 'recognisable entity', and the textbook *Cutaneous Adipose Tissue*, which he has co-authored, looks at the regulation of adipose tissue and the cellulite phenomenon in some detail.

Fat – Or Not?

Cellulite is frequently dismissed by sceptics, usually male, as being no different from ordinary fat. This is simply unobservant. Assume it was just 'fat'; why then does it afflict women who are of average weight or even underweight, with figures of otherwise normal proportions? There is no question that cellulite often accompanies excess fat in the body, but it is not synonymous with it. Cellulite arises among the fat cells, in the layer of fatty (or adipose) tissue beneath the skin, especially on the upper legs and buttocks, where women tend to store their reserves of fat. It can also settle around the knees and upper arms.

This tendency to collect in concentrated zones and pockets is one feature which distinguishes cellulite from ordinary fat, which is normally distributed evenly over the body. It also looks and feels quite different. Cellulite gives the skin a puckered appearance, whereas fat is smooth-surfaced. The reason for this is that healthy fat cells are able to move about freely, whereas the fat cells which form part of a cellulite condition are trapped in clusters within the connective tissue.

Unlike fat, cellulite cannot be shifted by reducing diets or exercise alone, as countless women can testify. The pounds may disappear and the muscle tone improve, but the tell-tale pits and bulges still remain. Dr Yvon Gall, a member of the Institut de Recherche Pierre Fabre, explains why: 'A fat cell is like a factory. Its speciality is to store fatty acids in some conditions and to release them in others. This depends on the activities of the workers in the cell, the enzymes. Cellulite is directly due to modified enzyme activity.'

In other words, the normal process of fat cells, releasing their stores of fatty acids during dieting and exercise, is prevented from happening by the action of an enzyme, in this case lipase. Instead you get abnormal fat storage, especially in women who are sensitive to oestrogen, which results in the formation of cellulite.

There are other differences too. The body needs a certain amount of fat – it provides us with the energy reserves to survive in hard times and enables the body to carry out a small number of important functions. It also allows a woman to sustain a pregnancy and nurture a young infant, irrespective of external conditions. Cellulite, on the other hand, does not have an 'up' side. It is a manifestation of a problem: internal pollution. The places in the body where cellulite most commonly occurs are the places where the body's unwanted wastes, the toxins that overtax the system, are dumped in fatty tissue to minimise the damage that they can cause.

Dumping Ground

Holistic GP Richard James believes that fat deposits absorb poisonous substances which the body cannot deal with, and contain them indefinitely. The knowledge that pesticide and herbicide residues detected in livestock are concentrated in their fat seems to bear this out. Dr James claims that all fat-soluble substances, including herbicides and pesticides, are naturally attracted to fatty tissue. This goes some way to explain why the toxins which enter the female body seem to make a bee-line for the hips and thighs.

The other theory is that the well-covered upper legs and rump provide safe storage for such substances away from the vital organs. But even in these so-called 'safe' locations, toxins cannot be entirely harmless – not if the lumps and bumps that result are anything to go by. The presence of cellulite broadcasts a clear message about the disturbance these impurities are causing in the system.

Cellulite and You

So how do you know if you have got cellulite? What are the main hallmarks? The acid test consists of squeezing the flesh on your upper thigh between your thumb and index finger. If cellulite is present, the texture will feel granular and lumpy, very much like cottage cheese. Beyond that, the intensity of symptoms varies enormously from one individual to the next. The 'orange peel' can be more or less visible depending on the age and weight of the individual, as well as the type of skin. The deep ripples and dimples of long-standing cellulite, however, speak for themselves.

Affected areas tend to be cooler and whiter than other flesh too. There are two reasons for this – fat is a poor conductor of heat, and congestion in the tissue beneath the skin restricts the flow of blood to the capillaries. Cellulite flesh also lacks the springiness of normal fatty tissue. One experienced aromatherapist compares the texture of the tissue in advanced cases to corrugated cardboard, others talk of strings of chipolatas and hard sago.

Really stubborn deposits often feel numb and the flesh quite coarse, due to the hardening of the tissue beneath. When inflammation and bloating occur in the tissue it can feel tender – even painful – to the touch. In some women this can be heightened by, or confined to, the days immediately before menstruation.

A Closer Look

The changes discernible to the eye and to touch have been described. But if the outer skin is registering such a disturbance, what is the picture beneath the surface? Structurally, the skin consists of three layers. The outer, thinner epidermis is a protective, waterproof layer responsible for generating new cells to replace the millions that die and are cast off daily. The inner, thicker part is called the dermis. It consists of different types of connective tissue which contain collagenous and elastic fibres, blood and lymph vessels, fine nerve endings and a ground substance in which they all sit. The triple spiral structure of collagen fibre gives the skin its strength, while the spring-like elastic fibres provide suppleness and stretchability.

Beneath the dermis is the subcutaneous layer, or hypodermis, which attaches the skin to the muscle and bone. This is the body's insulating layer and is composed of globules of fat cells, or adipocytes, set in loose connective tissue. The blood vessels and nerves also pass through the hypodermis. The walls which divide the dermis and the hypodermis are structured in such a way that groups of fat cells are able to move from the lower layer upwards into the dermis. This is what occurs during the process of cellulite formation.

Under the microscope, cellulite tissue reveals fat cells which are saturated with fluid and wastes and imprisoned in a fine network of hardened connective fibres. The walls of the fat cells are enveloped by extra deposits of collagen and soon develop into porridgy structures called 'micronodules'. These may later join together to form larger 'macronodules' which cause the uneven texture under the skin's surface. Nerve endings in the tissue also appear compressed.

—2—

What Causes Cellulite?

What are the physiological processes which bring about this unhealthy state of affairs? There are a number of predisposing factors which encourage cellulite to form. Poor circulation is chief among them. Blood, rich in oxygen and foodstuffs, provides nourishment for all the cells in the body. But an accumulation of wastes and water can interfere with that process, affecting microcirculation of blood and lymph. This is the thin end of the wedge for healthy tissue. An inadequate flow of blood to the capillaries which serve the fat cells means short rations of oxygen and nutrients, and only a partial removal of toxins via the lymphatic system. This results in stagnation in the tissue, and, almost inevitably, in some degree of cellulite.

Poor circulation often goes with a slow metabolism, but it can also have external causes. Wearing clothes which are too tight around the waist or the legs can constrict the blood flow. Hysterectomies, Caesarean sections and other pelvic operations can also interrupt the flow of blood and compromise the drainage of the tissues. This occurs usually because either blood and lymphatic vessels have been tied off in the course of the operation, or they are blocked and squeezed by the scar tissue that develops afterwards.

Poor elimination of the body's many waste products is bound to be a major factor, because it locks potentially harmful substances within the system. Underfunction of any of the eliminatory organs is obviously a serious handicap in this respect. But a condition as common as constipation, which can often go unrecognised, adds enormously to the body's rubbish load with its residue of undigested or partially digested foods. On top of the toxins in our diet, the impurities in our water and in the atmosphere and the by-products of the body's metabolic and regeneration processes, this adds up to a veritable mountain of waste. This is harboured throughout the body in organs, tissues, cells and in the spaces between the cells, known as interstitial spaces, containing a fluid which acts as a medium for the exchange of nutrients and wastes between the blood in the capillaries and the cells. Fatty tissue on the thighs, where the circulation is sluggish, is particularly prone to collecting waste because the exchange is less effective. This results in congestion, which takes its toll on the capillaries, causing their walls to weaken so that they start to seep blood plasma into the interstitial spaces. Eventually there is a serious build-up of fluid, which pushes cells and capillaries further apart and undermines the nutrient–waste exchange.

The accumulations of fat, toxins and fluids that result are, in effect, incipient bundles of cellulite. They migrate upwards into the dermis, the middle layer of skin tissue, where the fat cells clump into nodules. These nodules expand as layers of collagen fibres encapsulate their outer surface, until they represent sizeable masses, trapped in the fibrous tissue, compressing blood capillaries and compounding the congestion problem. And so cellulite is born.

The Lymphatic System

Our bodies are furnished with a rubbish-clearing system which has a critical role to play. It is called the lymphatic system and it works in tandem with, but independently from, the circulatory system, via a network of vessels of graduating size. The tiny capillaries, or 'lymphatics', in the subcutaneous tissue drain the liquid debris from the interstitial spaces and transport what is then called 'lymph', via strategically placed lymph nodes towards the lymphatic ducts in the upper body. The ducts filter the lymph before returning it via the heart to the bloodstream, so it can be further processed by the eliminative organs such as the liver and kidneys.

The smooth functioning of the lymphatic system is not automatic, as research carried out at the Université Libre in Brussels has clearly shown. Tests on women suffering from cellulite revealed that 100 per cent were affected by poor lymphatic drainage. The difference between blood and lymphatic circulation is that the lymph does not have a powerful pump like the heart to drive it. The movement of lymph towards the heart depends partly on the compression of lymphatic vessels by the muscles in our limbs, and partly on a siphon effect created by the action of respiration.

What is more, the left and right sides of the body are not equally well served by the two main collecting ducts of the lymphatic system. While the right lymphatic duct, which is located just inside the right collarbone, is only required to pool lymph from the upper right side of the body, the thoracic duct in the chest has to drain lymph from the left side of the head, neck and chest, the left arm and the entire body below the ribs. It is interesting to note that, almost without exception, cellulite is markedly more pronounced on the right leg than the left. It may be because the waste from that region has to take a long and circuitous route to the relevant filtering station without the benefit of a forceful mechanism to help it.

A Gender Issue

Why is it, then, that men are not blighted by the problem of cellulite? What is it about the female body that makes it such a fertile breeding ground? Dr Terence Ryan observes that the female tendency to develop cellulite, which can be passed on from mother to daughter in the genes and can even be activated in the womb, is strongly linked to anatomical type. There is a particularly high incidence of cellulite in 'pear-shaped' and Rubenesque women with large breasts and well-rounded figures (bad news for the British and the Afro-Caribbean female). Women with slow metabolisms, who put on weight easily and lose it with difficulty, are also especially prone.

There are other anatomical features which tip the balance against women. They have twice the amount of fatty tissue than men, which, given the principal part played by fat in the cellulite saga, does stack the odds against them. Lower levels of collagen in women's skin also result in thinner tissue, which makes the cellulite more apparent. In addition, the tissue on female thighs is more loosely structured and therefore more easily disrupted by the toxin and fluid build-up.

Age is another factor. As women get older, they experience a progressive thinning and breaking down of the connective tissue. The elasticity of the skin diminishes too over the years, or earlier if we are very inactive or overweight; even the most carefully preserved septuagenarian cannot have the firm flesh of a teenager. This fact has a direct bearing on the skin's ability to withstand internal disruption from a relatively early age – a fact substantiated by the reduced level of elastic fibres detected in cellulite tissue under the microscope.

Sun, pollution, smoking, stress and illness all have a prema-ture ageing effect which can hasten these changes. So can poor eating habits, especially inadequate protein intake and repeated dieting. The restrictions inherent in most diets inevitably reduce the level of essential nutrients the body is receiving. This means less nourishment for all the cells, including the skin cells. Crash diets, and the rapid weight loss which they encour-age, put the skin under further strain as it is forced to contract to deal with sudden reductions in bulk, only to have to expand again as the weight is piled back on. Extreme diets often fail to achieve the desired effect of burning up fat, and instead burn up the supporting muscle tissue.

It is not that men are immune to the risks presented by the dangers of excess weight and internal pollution, it is just that they deal with it in a different way. For one thing, they store their fat in a different place – usually around the midriff and closer to the vital organs. Although they are rarely troubled by the 'orange peel' phenomenon in that area, they do suffer a relatively higher incidence of heart disease up to middle age. This is the age when women's bodies are subject to the full range of hormonal activity and are busily transporting the risky substances to safe outposts, giving rise to cellulite.

Female Hormones

So women's bodies are programmed to function differently to men's. The instructions come from hormones, chemical messengers in the blood, whose job it is to alter the physiological activity of specific cells of the body.

It is the female sex hormones which are responsible for the development of breasts, underarm and pubic hair and the typically feminine proportions of the body. These include the fat deposits which start to appear on hips, thighs and shoulders from puberty onwards. Oestrogen and progesterone are the main players and they regulate the menstrual cycle and maintain pregnancy; or they can prevent it when the hormones are taken in a synthetic form via the contraceptive pill. They also interact with aldosterone (a hormone shared by both sexes) to control the fluid balance.

Over the last sixty years or so, French research has revealed a number of key facts about the nature of cellulite. The identification of water retention as the heart of the problem has been one of the most important. Since cellulite appeared to be an almost exclusively female complaint, scientists also began to examine possible links with hormonal activity. The realisation that oestrogen predisposes women to retain fluid was the final piece in the jigsaw. Whenever there is a burst of sex hormones, the body is programmed to store fat for later use – in pregnancy or for breastfeeding. But the poor circulation which is associated with fatty tissue means the area becomes a bit of a dead-end and fluids build up which cannot be released.

It seems that hormonal activity, which during certain phases in a woman's life can raise oestrogen to excessive levels, is a powerful trigger for the onset of cellulite and may be the principal cause in 75 percent of cases: 12 percent are believed to coincide with puberty, when the ovaries first become active and oestrogen production starts; 17 percent with pregnancy, which demands an increased supply of oestrogen and progesterone and can be accompanied by extra weight gain and poor circulation; and 27 percent in the run-up to the menopause, when progesterone production falls, again sending oestrogen levels out of balance. The body is especially vulnerable during these periods, so extra care is needed to limit other possible contributing factors such as poor diet and lack of exercise.

A further 19 percent of cellulite conditions are linked to oral contraceptives, particularly the high-dose pill, which is more inclined to lead to water retention and weight gain. Practitioners with a broad experience of treating cellulite would certainly add hormone replacement therapy (HRT), more accurately termed oestrogen replacement therapy, to the list of catalysts.

It is not surprising to learn that cellulite can take root or dramatically worsen after a miscarriage or termination, when the body has to dispose of an influx of hormones which suddenly become superfluous. The trauma and stress of such an event can have an impact on a range of body systems, including the nervous system, with far-reaching effects.

THE ROLE OF STRESS

There is a gland called the hypothalamus, also known as the 'master gland', which connects the nervous system and the hormone or endocrine system, the two major control systems of the body. When an individual is subjected to stress, sensors detect changes in the body's chemistry, temperature and blood pressure, as well as emotional shifts. These messages stimulate the hypothalamus to initiate, directly or indirectly, a whole range of responses, including the release of the hormone adrenaline and an increase in the blood sugar level, to deal with a perceived emergency.

Repeated stress is extremely wearing on the body and creates a disturbance in the internal environment. The hypothalamus acts to inhibit certain processes during stress, with such side-effects as water retention and high blood pressure. The energy which is made available to the body in the form of blood sugar is not needed, so it gets laid down on the thighs as fat. Prolonged stress can also disrupt normal eating patterns, induce sugar cravings and interfere with digestion, waste elimination and breathing. The muscular tension caused by stress inhibits nutrient–waste exchange in the tissues. Stress needs to be managed actively in order to minimise these adverse effects.

A Positive Approach

In the battle against cellulite, such biological factors as the anatomical make-up we are born with and the fluctuating levels of natural chemicals in our blood are beyond our control – it is a question of working within the possibilities. However, there *are* lifestyle choices which we can and should take responsibility for, because they can either undermine or enhance our capacity to deal with the everyday business of surviving and remaining healthy. It is clear that, although the body is remarkably adept at coping without any extra assistance from us, it can only sustain the effort for so long before its systems start to break down.

What We Eat

One of the areas of life where we do have almost total control is diet. In some ways this is an onerous responsibility. What we take into our bodies has a profound influence on our general well-being and the healthy state of our tissues. It is also of critical importance if you are trying to get rid of cellulite – and prevent it recurring in the future. Toxins, substances which can be poisonous to the body, place an unnecessary extra burden on a system already fully occupied with normal levels of waste.

So how do we know what is safe and what isn't? Regrettably, the food we take in from day to day, which satisfies our hunger and permits us to go about our business, does not necessarily enhance our health. External appearances are deceptive when even the most succulent-looking fresh produce can be loaded with the residues of pesticides, herbicides and fungicides used in modern farming methods. Arming yourself with a few basic food facts will serve as useful ammunition as you try and pick your way through the bewildering choice of foods available. Once you know what to look out for and what to avoid, you will become expert at reading labels and spotting the hidden toxins.

THE OLD ROGUES
We are only too familiar with the worst offenders. Caffeine, alcohol and nicotine are all highly toxic and destructive substances, which infiltrate the system and create the conditions for cellulite to flourish. They act as stimulants, pepping us up when we feel lethargic and underpowered, and they are often consumed in response to stress. Like all stimulants, they are potent and can be addictive. But the real danger comes when we

start to rely on them to supply us with energy, rather than looking to the sort of food which will sustain us properly and supply our body with the nutrients it needs.

Caffeine

It becomes a vicious circle. Every time you consume a caffeinated drink – and tea has only marginally lower levels than coffee – you experience an adrenaline surge which is no different to the 'fight or flight' reaction sparked off by real physical danger or an emotional trauma. However, as your body soon discovers, it is a false alarm, and so it cuts off the adrenaline supply and, suffering from the withdrawal symptoms, you fall into a slump, which very probably leaves you gasping for another injection of caffeine. If this is a familiar pattern in your life, then it is time to take steps to break it.

Alcohol

Alcohol, especially spirits, is a very concentrated source of fuel as well as being a poison in the body. Consumed in excess, it ends up surplus to requirements in the fat stores. Like caffeine, alcohol produces energy by increasing the level of glucose in the bloodstream, albeit via a different process.

The toxic effect of alcohol is very quick to penetrate the system. When you take a sip of alcohol, it immediately enters the bloodstream via the intestine and is then swiftly transported to the cells. Tolerance varies from one individual to the next, but is demonstrably lower in women than in men. The adverse effects of alcohol have a considerable bearing on cellulite formation: it depletes stores of essential fats and vitamin C, so essential to healthy skin, and taxes that bastion of detoxification, the liver. It also hampers cellular exchange.

Also, if you drink wine, you may find your grape is laced with an unhealthy dose of colourings, flavourings and pesticides, unless it is organic.

Nicotine

It should not be necessary to enumerate the many dangers of tobacco smoking to our health, but the sobering facts are that smokers dramatically reduce their life expectancy; lung, throat and mouth cancer or some form of lung or coronary heart disease are the most common causes of death. Cigarettes are tubes of concentrated poison, and the act of smoking does nothing but damage, distributing carcinogenic substances, unleashing dangerous free radicals, consuming valuable vitamins and starving healthy blood cells of precious oxygen. Pale complexions and premature facial lines speak volumes about the adverse effects on smokers' skin.

It seems that the toxins which we misguidedly take into our bodies do not just overload our eliminative organs and throw our internal environment out of kilter, they can also contribute to serious disease processes. But these are the demons that we are continuously warned against and therefore, in theory, better equipped to resist. There is a whole galaxy of foods, with dubious benefits and increasingly publicised dangers, which we are consuming in alarming quantities.

Fat in food

Fat accounts for up to 40 percent of the calorie intake in the UK, at least twice the recommended maximum. In fact, it is reckoned that a healthy adult requires no more than 5g of fat a day to carry out the body's various fat-related functions. Fat consumption is incontrovertibly linked with obesity and heart disease. Due to its mucus-forming nature, fat also appears to present an obstacle to smooth digestion and elimination.

Fats fall into two categories: the saturated fats, and the polyunsaturated or monounsaturated fats. The high-risk saturated fats, generally of animal origin, are present in very high proportions in dairy products and red meat, and are a significant but often overlooked ingredient in pastries, pies and most processed foods. Polyunsaturated and monounsaturated fats tend to originate from plants and present far fewer risks to health, although they are not hazard free.

Fatty foods are also cellulite-forming foods. Their sticky wastes move slowly through the digestive system, leaving behind a residue which makes conditions difficult for the foods that follow. The cumulative effect is that wastes get trapped in the intestine, causing toxins to be reabsorbed into the blood, while the coating on the intestine walls makes the channel ever narrower and blocks the uptake of nutrients. Even the lymph takes on the viscous quality of fatty substances, which further hampers elimination at cell level.

One of the most toxic threats to the body comes from heated fats. The heating process changes their chemical structure and releases destructive particles called free radicals. Free radicals can seriously damage cell structures – they seem particularly to target cell membranes and both collagen and elastin proteins – and they actively precipitate the ageing and degenerating process in the skin and body as a whole. A scientific link has been established between free radicals and both cancer and heart disease caused by hardening of the arteries.

Allergy-causing foods

Both dairy products and wheat are common sources of allergy these days. Amongst the allergic responses which they can produce is, paradoxically, a craving for the food which disagrees. Eating allergenic foods can also encourage fluid retention as the body attempts to dilute the substance once it has entered the system. This bloating, known as allergic oedema, can be triggered by any food which the body cannot tolerate. Needless to say, this reaction aggravates the problems faced by the cellulite sufferer.

Intolerance to apparently innocuous foods (which may be staples in the diet) can also develop, precisely because consumption of them is so high. Wheat, one of the most overused ingredients in our diet, falls into this category – it is also one of the most common causes of constipation.

Sugar and salt

Sugar and salt are, as stimulants, hardly less addictive and harmful to the system than the more obvious substances. Sugar must surely be the ultimate non-nutrient. Although it is capable of supplying us with energy, it is an undesirable source, loading us up with useless calories and bringing tooth decay and obesity in its wake. Rather worryingly, our average annual consumption is estimated at a kilo a week.

The role of sugar – and salt for that matter – in the late twentieth-century diet is that of seducer and corrupter. The food scientists and marketing wizards are only too aware of the addictive qualities of both of these staple additives which they use without restraint in order to get your taste buds hooked. You only have to read the labels on the packets to see that. Both substances trigger reactions which bring about a temporary increase in energy and well-being, followed by the inevitable droop.

The level of salt (or sodium) in the body has an important role to play in regulating fluids. Sodium works with the mineral potassium to balance the fluid content, and an excess of salt threatens the all-important sodium–potassium balance both inside and outside the cells, encouraging fluid retention in the tissues. This waterlogging, always intensified around hips and thighs, creates optimum conditions for tissue congestion to occur, and for cellulite to flourish.

Junk

The last word must be reserved for 'junk' food – it has an awful lot to answer for. Over the centuries man has adapted to dietary changes without calamitous consequences. However, the advent of 'junk'(or processed or convenience) food seems to have done more harm than any single other change so far. While the huge list of additives and preservatives may produce a successful product that keeps the consumer coming back for more, it totally destroys the value of the majority of the ingredients used. In other words, nutritionally speaking this food is a pale shadow of its former self.

More importantly, we are now taking in, via both processed and 'pure' foods, a frightening quantity and variety of chemical substances for which our body has not evolved a way of dealing with. In addition to the chemicals showered over fruit and vegetables, most of our meat is contaminated by residues of the steroids, hormones and antibiotics fed routinely to livestock. Because the body cannot process them, it has to store them. Inevitably, some of them end up in the poor old thighs, leaving a trail of destruction behind them as they pass through the system. Dr Elisabeth Dancey, a London GP who treats cellulite, sums up the problem: 'We can't metabolise artificial things. We don't have the enzymes to deal with them, so they just hang around like a spanner in the works.'

3

Anti-Cellulite Tactics

Before you embark on an anti-cellulite regime it is important to tell yourself that you *can* beat cellulite without having to resort to painful and expensive cosmetic surgery. It will require a lot of determination and staying power and there may be times when you feel thoroughly fed up with the whole project, but do not lose sight of the fact that you have it in you to achieve the results you want. Think forward to a time when you can feel proud of your body and at ease in whatever clothes you wish to wear. Imagine a summer when you do not dread the idea of being seen in a swimsuit, and can pull on a pair of shorts or wear the sheerest tights without a second thought.

You may have accumulated a wardrobe full of clothes which are a little longer, fuller and maybe darker than you would like to choose, but which have done an admirable job in camouflaging a bottom-heavy silhouette. Perhaps you have even written off clothes which you are convinced you have 'outgrown'. Be prepared for a pleasant surprise – but be realistic. You cannot change your basic body type or the size of your bones. However, there is a lot you can do to remodel the flesh that shapes it and undo the damage which has caused it to sag, dimple and bulge.

The Bottom Line

As the weeks progress, you will be able to watch as the lines of your body are resculptured and the lumps and bumps, which you had begun to assume were meant to be there, gradually disappear. Needless to say, these sorts of changes do not occur overnight, nor will they happen without a great deal of effort on your part.

We have seen that the causes of cellulite are numerous, and the build-up cumulative. Hormones, stress, dietary and other indiscretions, as well as lifestyle habits, will all have played their part over the years, or decades, gradually adding to the cellulite burden. Time and an all-encompassing approach are what are now required to undo the damage.

This may mean a radical rethink of your diet, your exercise routine (or lack of it) and a new strategy to deal with the pressures in your life. If you stand back, you may be able to see the factors in your lifestyle which have contributed to the problem. It is up to you to reverse those trends and adopt a fresh approach which will tackle the problem from without and within.

Your immediate aim is to spring-clean your overburdened system, while setting your sights on the longer-term goal of limiting the build-up of toxins in the future. It may seem like an enormous undertaking, but the rewards are huge and extend far beyond reclaiming your smooth, cellulite-free body. You will find yourself with greater stores of energy and buoyed up by your improved self-esteem. Your perspective on life will seem clearer and your emotions steadier. Increased vitality will probably make you less susceptible to colds and other ailments too.

The Hard Truth About Diet

The fact is that your body can only take so much abuse. Unfortunately, the 'modern' diet – a far cry from the natural wholefood diet of our ancestors – is a minefield for the cellulite sufferer because of its high sugar and fat content and emphasis on refined and processed foods. The human body does not thrive on these substances; in fact, it is positively polluted by them. The liver, kidneys and bowel are equipped to process and eliminate toxins and waste up to a certain level. Once they reach their capacity, the only alternative is for those substances to remain in the system.

We have already named some of the toxins implicated in the formation of cellulite – caffeine, nicotine and alcohol being among the worst culprits. If you start to add undesirable quantities of salt, sugar and saturated fat plus a liberal dose of additives and preservatives, it is not hard to see how your system could soon start to suffer under the strain. Cellulite is an external manifestation of that internal overload.

In order to function optimally, the body needs to be fuelled by a cocktail of nutrients derived from the food we consume. That means making sure that we have a balanced diet, containing the right ratio of proteins, carbohydrates, fats, fresh fruit and vegetables. These provide us with enough energy to go about our daily business (plus a little extra to store away), as well as the wherewithal to maintain and repair our bodies. By taking care to feed our bodies the right things, we also protect the all-important chemical balance in our internal environment.

That said, it is all too easy to stray from the golden path. Whether it is out of convenience, or a result of social pressures, time pressures, stress or sheer indulgence, our diet starts to lose its balance and our general health deteriorates in the process. Identifying the foods which encourage cellulite and prejudice a healthy internal environment is the first step in the right direction.

As far as your diet is concerned, the objective is to cut out the foods which do not bring the body any benefits and cut down on the foods which interfere with the uptake of nutrients and the elimination of wastes. These need to be replaced with health-enhancing foods which work for you rather than against you. You need to rid the body of the rubbish which has been allowed to build up as a result of sloppy habits or ignorance. These must be banished as a first step towards conquering cellulite.

The best way to achieve this is by spring-cleaning your insides with a special cleansing or detoxification regime (see Chapter 4). This could take a number of courses depending on your general state of health and the condition of your heart, liver and kidneys. Diabetics and pregnant women are advised against embarking on such a regime. It is important to consult your doctor to get the safe go-ahead. Another book of mine, the *Quick Guide to Detox* (Boxtree), explains detoxification in detail.

The Hard Truth About Exercise

A sedentary lifestyle is a major factor in the formation of cellulite. Sitting or standing in one position for extended periods of time during your working and leisure hours will, inevitably, result in slower circulation and an underactive metabolism. Dermatologist Dr Terence Ryan warns against the ageing effect on the skin if flesh is 'allowed to get weighty, obese and cold'. Exercise has therefore to be an essential component of the cellulite-beating regime.

By encouraging deeper breathing and galvanising sluggish circulation and lymphatic drainage, exercise can actually help with the elimination of excess fluid and toxins which accumulate in tissue spaces. It also speeds up the rate at which we burn fat, even when we are not exercising, and discourages the digestive system from retaining harmful material. However, in order to be effective, it must be regular.

If you can, build exercise into your daily routine. Everybody knows that it does them no end of good to walk up stairs rather than taking the escalator or lift and that it is sheer laziness that makes us drive a short distance when we could easily walk. This does not stop us from taking the easy option. If you cannot change your working conditions, you may need to redouble your efforts outside work. When it comes to building your exercise programme, try to choose an activity which you positively enjoy. That way you are more likely to make an effort to fit it into a busy schedule.

EVERY LITTLE HELPS

If you like gardening, then do it regularly and with vigour. If you own a bicycle, make sure it is roadworthy and use it for local errands or consider whether you could cycle to work. Dancing is one of the best forms of exercise – the more energetic the better.

Take every opportunity that comes your way to tone your muscles and get your heart beating a little faster. Whatever you do will make a difference. Use the time which would otherwise be spent sitting still in front of the television to practise a few exercises or relax with some deep breathing. You can also assist the flow of lymph from the hip and thigh area by lying with your legs raised on the arm of a sofa or by bicycling in the air for a few minutes every day.

AEROBIC IS BEST

Different types of exercise have different effects on the body's physique and internal workings. The sort of exercise which is right for fighting cellulite is low-intensity aerobic exercise which improves your general fitness by improving the performance of your heart and lungs and burning up excess fat and calories. In order to maximise the benefits of exercise, you need to aim to exercise for twenty minutes or more, at 60 percent of your maximum heart rate, at least three times a week.

First of all, you need to calculate your maximum heart rate (MHR), which is very simple, especially if you have a calculator to hand. First take your pulse, by pressing down on the artery at the wrist with three fingers and counting the number of heartbeats that occur over six seconds. Then multiply this figure by ten to calculate your resting heart rate. To work out your maximum heart rate, subtract your age from 220. Multiply this figure by 0.6 (or 60 percent), and you have your target heart rate (THR). So, if you are thirty years old:

MHR = 220 - 30 = 190 beats per minute (BPM)
THR = 190 BPM x 60 percent = 114 BPM

THE BENEFITS

During exercise, your heart is encouraged to pump more blood round the system, sending extra supplies to the skin to help release excess heat produced by muscular action. Increased blood flow provides the cells in the sluggish subcutaneous tissue of the hips and thighs with fresh nutrients and removes stagnant wastes, literally breathing new life into 'deadened' areas. At the same time, the cells are stimulated to release fatty acids and turn them into energy, helping to reduce the stockpile on thighs and hips.

Your skeleton changes its position too. As your muscles gently stretch and relax, a natural pressure is created which helps the lymphatic system to carry out its job of bodily cleansing. And apart from literally shaking you out of your torpor, exercise has the potential to lift your spirits, release tension and help you see things in a different perspective.

Brisk walking or cycling in 'quality' air are especially recommended, as they give your body a gentle but thorough workout. Walking, especially on grass, is one of the safest and most effective ways to achieve all-round fitness. The action of walking effectively squeezes and stretches the digestive tract and promotes good muscle tone in abdominal muscles and throughout the digestive system.

Swimming has the advantage of toning muscles and improving cardiovascular condition without placing any strain on the joints, while the resistance of the water ensures that your muscles are forced to work harder in every direction. An energetic crawl, backstroke or butterfly will get your heart pumping faster than a sedate breast stroke.

You could also slip in a few underwater hip and thigh toners at the end of your swimming session:

* For the bottom. Stand sideways to the pool wall and hold on to the side. Keeping your back straight and your left foot flat on the floor, lift and bend your right knee towards the chest. Straighten your leg out in front of you. Slowly swing the straight leg backwards until you feel the buttocks 'squeeze'. Repeat five–ten times on each leg.

* For the inner and outer thighs. Stand sideways to the pool wall and lift the outer leg to the side as far as possible. Sweep the leg forwards so that it crosses in front of the supporting leg. Sweep the leg out again. Repeat the movement, swinging the leg backwards. Repeat five–ten times on each leg.

* Finish up by striding as far as you can up the pool and back again, using your arms to help propel you.

Any exercise you can do in the fresh air (preferably away from main roads or other obvious sources of pollution) will bring extra benefits. A daily dose of fresh air feeds your cells, ensures a fresh supply of oxygen to the brain and exercises your internal organs, as well as ridding your body of excess carbon dioxide.

During the spring-clean, sleep with windows open (add extra blankets if necessary) to allow your body to continue the beneficial process at night.

THE BREATH OF LIFE

It is a good idea to spend some time focusing on your breathing. We have mentioned the role that breathing plays in lymphatic circulation. Most of us use only half of our capacity to take in oxygen and expel carbon dioxide. We would reap huge benefits if we could inhale and exhale to our full capacity.

In order to do this, you need to develop abdominal breathing, instead of concentrating the effort in the chest. Try to take more time over each breath, inhaling until your lungs have had their fill of oxygen and exhaling slowly and fully, pausing with the natural lull before allowing the next breath to arise. It will boost the lymph flow immeasurably and induce a feeling of calm.

THE G-FORCE

Rebounding on a mini-trampoline (or bouncer) is another option, believed by some to be the best possible form of exercise for combating cellulite because of the use it makes of the force of gravity. The up-and-down movement, which first suspends your body in space and then subjects it to two or three times the force of gravity, stimulates the elimination of wastes through your lymph system. Increased oxygen is also brought to the cells, boosting the whole system and encouraging gradual detoxification.

The great appeal of rebounding is that you can do it in the privacy of your own home, at your own convenience, irrespective of your age, your level of fitness or of the weather outside. You can bounce to music, while you listen to the radio or in front of the television. You can even skip at the same time. Ten minutes at the beginning of the day will really kick-start your system. A vigorous session in the early evening will maximise the rest of the day and dispel any feelings of lethargy or stress that may be weighing you down. Another benefit is that you will never be troubled by constipation while you are rebounding regularly.

DON'T OVERDO IT

Within these guidelines, moderation is still the watchword. Exercise is meant to enhance your body, not injure it. Do what is comfortable and gradually increase the time and effort rather than setting yourself punishing targets.

The golden rule is that if you feel any strain or discomfort – stop.

Also give some thought to your posture. The alignment of your spine, the central channel of the nervous system, is inextricably linked to the flow of energy within your body. When you break your posture, say by sticking out your bottom, the spine is not working as a unit, and the energy flow is disturbed. High heels throw your posture out of line by pitching the body weight forwards. Good posture, which instantly improves the figure, is about thinking tall. So, lift up from your pelvis, tuck in your tailbone, extend your spine and drop your shoulders. Go through those motions as often as you remember to until they become second nature.

Yoga is an exercise form which focuses on breathing and posture as well as developing the art of relaxation. Regular practice can remove blockages caused by tension and stiffness, especially around the sacrum, the triangular base of the spine which forms part of the pelvis. This sort of blockage can affect the supply of oxygen and disposal of wastes in the lower body. The shoulder stand, one of the core yoga positions, is a superb therapy for the lymphatic system. Like most forms of exercise, yoga has psychological benefits as well.

TONING ROUTINE

Devote at least ten minutes a day to conditioning your body with the specially targeted toning exercises described below. If you do not exercise your muscles, they lose their tone and start to become a liability. Firm muscle provides better support for tissue than flabby muscle. The effects of poor muscle tone are specifically linked to cellulite.

You can see how muscle condition can contribute to a cellulite problem if you look at the gluteus maximus muscles in the buttocks. When they are toned and taut, they prevent the buttocks from weighing down on the upper thighs, adding pressure to an area that may already be encumbered by excess fat and fluid. The stomach muscles, if they are allowed to get lazy, can lead to poor posture and interfere with lymphatic drainage. The inner thighs are especially prone to cellulite because the muscles are so often allowed to become slack, which turns them into a collecting pool for stagnant waste and water.

* *Thigh shaper and tummy tightener.* Sit on the floor with your lower back against a wall. Open your legs, bend your knees and place your finger tips on the floor in front of you. Lean on your hands and raise both legs, then straighten and stretch your legs and really point your toes. Relax. Repeat three times, gradually increasing to eight as your muscles get stronger. As you get stronger, try to bend and straighten your legs a few times while keeping your legs in the air. This exercise may seem very hard to begin with, but do persist – it produces fantastic results.

* *Inner thigh squeeze.* Lie flat on your back and bend your knees, keeping your feet flat on the floor and hip-width apart. Place a cushion or football between

your inner thighs and inch your feet closer together. Press your lower back into the floor, holding your abdominal muscles firm. Slowly squeeze the whole length of your inner thighs together and then relax. Breathe easily throughout. Repeat ten times, working up to thirty.

* *Inner thigh stretch.* Sit on the floor with your back straight and your knees bent with the soles of your feet together. Breathe in, and on the out-breath push your knees down towards the floor. Repeat, releasing your knees further with each out-breath.

* *Bottom and back thigh toner.* Lie on your tummy and rest your chin on the floor. Place your hands by your side with palms down. Open legs wide and raise both legs off the floor, with knees very slightly bent. Now with little pushes from the thighs, open your legs wider. Keep pushing open then hold. Relax and repeat twice more.

Your Skin

In addition to the necessary modifications to your diet and exercise regime, there are several other simple but effective ways in which you can help your body to dispose of accumulated rubbish and reverse the stagnation process in the cells and tissues of vulnerable areas. The skin is an important organ of elimination along with the lungs, the colon and the kidneys. Sometimes referred to as the 'third kidney', it is, in fact, the largest of the four eliminative organs and discharges more than 1lb a day in waste products via its thousands of sweat glands and two million or so pores. This vital function helps to reduce the level of harmful waste, which in turn reduces susceptibility to cellulite.

However, if the skin becomes inactive because the pores are clogged with dead cells, it is unable to do its job properly and uric acid (one of the main constituents of sweat) and other impurities remain trapped in the system. Regular baths and showers help to keep pores clear by washing away the dead skin cells, but this may not be enough. When the body's levels of accumulated toxins reach a certain point, the eliminative organs are under increased pressure to clear the debris, and benefit from extra assistance.

BRUSHING FOR HEALTH

Dry skin brushing is an easy and inexpensive way to achieve this. Using friction and a form of acupressure, the bristles act directly on the lymph vessels and capillaries to stimulate the lymph and blood circulation to remove impurities from under the skin's surface. It is important to remember that lymph circulates slowly and against gravity. By encouraging the flow towards the lymph nodes (or filtering stations) and ultimately towards the heart, where the largest collection of nodes is located, you will improve the efficiency of lymphatic drainage.

Devotees claim a catalogue of benefits from skin brushing, ranging from improved skin texture, renewed energy levels and a general sense of well-being, to better digestion and a more efficient metabolism. It also thoroughly exfoliates the skin in preparation for the application of anti-cellulite oils or creams.

At the beginning, it seems rather a peculiar and disagreeable thing to inflict on yourself. The brush feels rough against your skin and your body tingles and smarts when it makes contact with water. After a few weeks of religious brushing, by which time you and your hide have acclimatised, you will regard this invigorating ritual as a fair exchange for the peachy skin that you will possess. Here are a few tips to get you started.

You need to get hold of a natural bristle brush with a long detachable handle. A soft brush or loofah will not produce the same results. Remember that this is *dry* skin brushing so get into the habit of doing it before your bath or shower. On wet skin the bristles will drag without creating the necessary friction. The routine should take no more than five minutes – maybe slightly longer while you are learning the ropes. Aim to do it daily for the first couple of months and then every other day. Make it a permanent feature of your bathing routine if you want to discourage cellulite formation in the future.

The method is to work from your extremities towards your heart using long, firm strokes. You should aim to brush over every section twice. Starting at your fingertips, brush the palms and backs of your hands then move up your arms, wrist to elbow, elbow to shoulder. Then do your feet, brushing over the soles, across the toes, round the ankles and up to the knee. Brush over the backs of the knees and then home in on the main cellulite zone, the upper leg. You may want to take a little longer over this and vary your upwards strokes to include some circular movements over the outer thighs and buttocks.

A gentle clockwise motion is ideal over the abdomen. Do not forget to brush up the sides of your body and the lower back, where toxins can easily collect. Stop once you are level with the heart and move up to the chin. Brush down the neck to the breastbone and then work round to your right and left earlobe allowing your strokes to radiate down over your breasts just short of your nipples, and outwards to the tips of your shoulder and over your upper back. Finally, rotate the brush gently on the inner side of your armpit towards your breast where the important axillary nodes are located. You should not brush quite so vigorously the tender areas of skin covering the neck, chest and stomach.

Always brush your body using long, firm strokes in the direction of the heart.

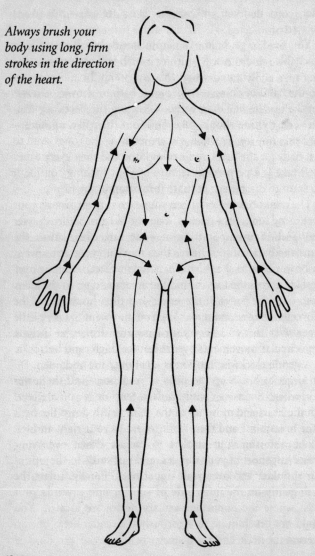

A word or two of warning. Avoid bruised, broken, inflamed or infected skin. If you suffer from eczema or psoriasis or have any varicose veins, do not brush near affected areas. If you find the brush intolerably rough, soak it in warm water then allow it to dry naturally overnight. In any case you will need to wash it every few weeks – probably once a week during the detoxification phase – for hygienic reasons. The odours that your brush will take up in the first few weeks are proof that something is being eliminated!

Hands-On Therapy

Massage is another valuable weapon in the battle against cellulite which can support your efforts on the diet and exercise front. Like skin brushing, it can speed up the general cleansing process by activating the return of blood to the heart and of lymph to the lymphatic ducts. Frequent massage in problem areas over a period of time can also whittle away stubborn deposits of cellulite and make connective tissue more supple.

Massage has the ability to melt away tension, calm jangled nerves and ease and relax muscles – which must make it almost compulsory in the pressured lives we all lead!

Lymphatic drainage massage is a treatment specifically recommended for cellulite breakdown, as the lymphatic system plays such an important part in controlling the toxic build-up in cells and tissues (see Chapter 4). Carried out by a trained professional, it can have a dramatic effect, improving the exchanges between cells and interstitial fluid and speeding up removal of cellular wastes. It is almost impossible to carry out on yourself.

DO-IT-YOURSELF
Any massage that you do perform will improve the flow of

blood round the body and therefore revitalise those deadened areas where cellulite tends to collect. The hand-to-skin contact causes the blood vessels beneath the surface to dilate which allows the blood to circulate more easily. Although professional treatment may be of particular use in tackling hard and long-standing cellulite deposits, you can nevertheless achieve a huge amount yourself by practising some techniques for five or ten minutes every day.

Self-massage will provide an opportunity for you to rediscover and lavish some attention on a part of your body you might have chosen to ignore. Pin-point the real trouble spots, because that is where your massaging efforts need to be focused. Do not punish your thighs with too much pummelling and pounding though; the fragile capillaries in cellulite-affected tissue need careful handling. Rhythmic, gentle movements and frequent repetition will achieve far more.

Bath-time, both in and out of the water, is the best time to massage. Add a few drops of stimulating and detoxifying essential oils (rosemary, juniper, fennel and cypress are all recommended) and a splash of plain oil and soak for fifteen minutes. Lying in the bath, you are in a good position to work on your upper legs, lifting and gently squeezing the flesh to release the trapped toxins. At first the more cellulite-ridden areas will feel very tender and resent being disturbed. Go easy and persevere. You will soon notice a change in texture as the hard nodules start to loosen up and the sensitivity begins to ease. You may even detect a 'popping' sensation.

You can continue the process when you get out of the bath, using an oil or lotion as a lubricant. You can make your own detoxing massage oil from a blend of essential oils mixed into a carrier or base oil. Grapeseed and almond oils are good bases to which you can add a few drops each of fennel, juniper, cypress and geranium essential oils. When using massage oil, tip a teaspoonful into the palm of your hand and rub your hands together before you begin. Glide the oil up the leg from the foot to the top of the thigh, using firm stroking movements to warm and relax the muscles. Then work the knee area, pressing as you rotate your thumbs in small circles. Make the hand into a fist and, pushing the knuckles into the thigh, move up the upper leg on the front, back, inside and outside of the thighs. You can then spend a little more time on the inner and outer thighs, massaging in towards the middle using wringing, rolling and kneading motions. It is also useful to vary your technique with horizontal, vertical and circular movements. Overvigorous massage can cause broken blood vessels to appear on the surface of the skin, in which case a gentler approach is required.

Baths in General

Make your daily bath a sacred ritual and use it to unwind and concentrate on your breathing as well as your body. Don't run a very hot bath – blood temperature is ideal, though it may be cooler than you are used to. Very hot baths can damage the skin by drying the outer layer and damaging the capillaries. For a soothing detoxifying bath, dissolve two handfuls of Epsom salts (also known as magnesium sulphate and available from chemists) and one handful of rock salt in running water and soak for a minimum of twenty minutes. This is useful early on in the regime – and after lapses.

You can increase blood flow to cellulite areas by subjecting them to a cold shower treatment when you have finished bathing. Paddling in cold water is a good remedy for poor circulation in general. It is particularly effective if you suffer from cold feet. Fill a bath ankle-high with cold water and walk up and down for at least a minute – longer if you can manage it. Be careful not to slip. When you get out, you will notice that your feet, contrary to what you would expect, are warmer than before. This is because the blood goes rushing to the extremities to counteract the cooling effects of the water.

Predictions and Results

Once you have begun to wage serious war on your cellulite, by looking at all of the relevant areas of your life and making the necessary changes, how long will it be before you can expect to see results and how dramatic will they be? Whether your cellulite disappears after six weeks or six months depends on how established it is. The cause of the cellulite will also determine the eventual outcome. In a few cases there are anatomical or physiological reasons why the body cannot prevent the congestion or waste levels which may encourage cellulite to form. In other cases, the contraceptive pill is the main cause of the cellulite which will never be tackled successfully while you continue to take it.

One thing is certain: the curve of progress will not necessarily be smooth and steady. There will be some weeks when you feel your efforts are being well rewarded and others when you wonder whether it is all worth-while. Keep reassuring yourself emphatically that it is. You are doing something for yourself which will have long-term benefits as well as short-term gratifications. The results, while they will be most noticeable on the outside, will have far greater impact on the inside, where it really counts.

——— 4 ———
The Anti-Cellulite Diet

How you go about detoxifying your system will depend on a number of factors. In addition to the health implications already discussed, the intensity of the detoxification programme will be dictated by existing levels of toxicity in the body, individual metabolism and the question of how fast you want to see results. There is also the problem of fitting the whole project around a busy working day or a demanding family.

People suffering from low blood sugar (and there are a surprising number) need to include a certain proportion of the more sustaining types of food in their diet from the outset to maintain blood sugar levels. This rules out a lengthy period on just fruit and vegetables. For some, however, the uncompromising fruit and vegetable regime is a very effective and powerful way to kick-start the cleansing process.

Most people considering a regime of this kind have a few skeletons in the cupboard in the form of dietary 'props' which need to be phased out before the serious business of detoxification can begin. Here's how to go about it.

First Steps

Start gradually to cut back on tea, coffee, cigarettes and alcohol. Try and limit yourself to one or two cups of tea and coffee a day and, if possible, make sure that the coffee you drink is freshly ground. Avoid instant coffee altogether. Investigate the full range of herbal teas and coffee substitutes available to find a few that you really like. The strange-sounding rooibosh tea is worth trying: it contains neither caffeine nor tannin and yet looks and tastes like Indian tea – you can also add milk to it. It's certainly a lot more appetising than most of the decaffeinated teas currently available.

The Danger Areas

Concentrate on developing a healthier way of eating by dramatically reducing your consumption of the following foods:

* *Fats.* In red meat and dairy products. Opt for lower-fat game, poultry and fish. Switch to semi-skimmed milk and low-fat cheeses. Heavy, hard cheeses are acidic as well as being very high in fat. Use butter (unsalted) very sparingly for cooking and spreading. Steam, grill or bake foods rather than frying. If you must fry, use cold-pressed extra virgin olive oil.

* *Processed foods,* ie all foods which have been altered in some way to increase their palatability or their shelf life. This includes fast food, pre-prepared sauces and meals, and preserved, frozen and canned foods.

* *Refined carbohydrates,* eg white flour, white bread, white pasta.

* *Sugar* – white and brown, syrup and treacle – has no use in the body, but it is very effective at rotting our teeth and swelling our fat stores. Honey has a slight edge only because of the vitamins, minerals and enzymes it contains. Try and wean yourself off sweet things, including artificially sweetened food. Look for

sugar-free pure fruit jams. Make puddings an
occasional treat.

* *Salt.* The best way to reduce the amount of salt in
your diet is to buy fresh food and prepare it yourself,
then at least you know how much you're taking in.
Try cutting out salt at the cooking stage but allow
yourself a pinch or two at the table, so that you really
taste it. Use sea salt only. Avoid salted snacks such as
crisps and peanuts.

Glorious Foods

Make these ingredients a priority in your diet:

* *Fresh fruit and vegetables.* Have a couple of pieces of
fruit as a mid-morning or mid-afternoon snack in
preference to pastries or biscuits. Incorporate a salad
into your lunch and evening meal, either as a starter, a
main course or a side vegetable. If you want to cook
vegetables, steam them lightly in a small amount of
water or bake them. Buy organic whenever possible
and always wash before eating.

* *Wholegrains.* Wholewheat bread, pastry and pasta,
brown rice, oats, rye, corn, couscous.

* Cultivate a taste for *natural yoghurt*, especially the
'live' variety. It is a health-giving food which helps
restore the healthy intestinal flora, often damaged by
eating a diet too high in refined foods.

* *Water.* You need to be aiming to drink one–two litres

of water per day, which may take a big conscious effort. The easiest way to do this is to carry a bottle around with you or have a glass permanently to hand so that you can sip away continuously. If you are not going to be drinking bottled water, then it is worth investing in a water filter jug which is also useful for larger quantities when cooking. Tap water may contain toxic metals and other contaminants.

Acid or Alkaline?

Another point to consider is the acid/alkaline balance of your food. You may not be aware that all foods end up as either alkaline or acid remains once they have been digested by the body. This does not necessarily correspond to the taste sensation detected by your palate. For instance, citrus fruits taste acid in the mouth, but are alkaline once they enter the bloodstream. This is important when you consider the alkalinity of our blood, maintained at a precise level of pH7.4. The minerals contained in alkaline-forming foods allow the blood to maintain its alkaline state.

Broadly speaking, proteins (meat, fish, poultry, eggs, cheese), grains and some nuts are acid forming while most fruits and vegetables, other nuts, milk and yoghurt are alkaline forming. The diet on which our hunter-gatherer ancestors flourished is believed to have been 60–80 percent alkaline forming. There is much evidence to suggest that it is a balance that our digestive system likes. You can emulate this by shifting the balance of the modern diet, estimated to be 95 percent acid forming, and treating the protein element of your meal as the icing on the cake.

The Question of Protein

Too much protein has a negative effect because the body has to do a lot of work to break it down. More waste products are produced from protein digestion than from any other type of food, which can cause a build-up of toxins if you are not eliminating them effectively from the bowel. Eating between 30 and 70 grams of protein a day is about right, depending on your weight, level of activity and your state of health.

However, protein, the body's main building material, has a very important part to play in the anti-cellulite diet. Without it, the body lacks the necessary resources to accomplish dozens of different processes, including the creation of new muscle and tissue. Fish is probably the healthiest source of complete protein, but vegetarians can combine nuts, seeds and grains with pulses to provide an equally nutritious alternative.

Once you have made these changes in your diet, thereby reducing the level of toxins in the system, you will be ready for the next stage of the regime. This involves following a natural wholefood diet, one which automatically excludes the foods that tax your system and promotes those foods capable of cleansing your body of old residue and loading it up with generous quantities of the nutrients it needs.

Raw Food

The emphasis is on raw fruit and vegetables as these have the capacity to speed up the process of elimination with a minimum of harmful effects. These natural and highly nutritious foods are very easily digested, which allows for the immediate uptake of vitamins and minerals into the body while expending the minimum amount of energy. This also frees up more energy to assist with the detoxification process itself. The fructose (fruit sugar) element will help to keep up your blood sugar level.

Cellulose, the natural fibre in raw fruit and vegetables, binds with waste in the digestive tract, while the high water content helps to flush out the system. Alkaline-forming fruit and vegetables can also help to neutralise stored wastes and toxins, which tend to be acidic in nature, as they are taken into the bloodstream. The high potassium content of fruit and vegetables has the effect of ridding the body of excess water and bringing sodium levels back into balance.

Eat your fruit and vegetables as fresh as possible, preferably within a day or two of buying them. Try to get hold of organic produce whenever you can. Fruit or vegetables which have been fed with chemical fertilisers and treated with pesticides, insecticides and fungicides will place an additional strain on your body as it tries to throw off the accumulated toxins.

However, if you cannot get hold of organic produce, don't worry. The worry will do more harm than the chemicals in the long run. Just remember to wash everything thoroughly before use. It is a good idea while you are detoxifying to soak non-organic produce for fifteen minutes in a solution of cider vinegar (three tablespoons of vinegar to one litre of water). Rinse and dry before eating.

Pep Talk

* Do not attempt this process during a busy period or when under undue stress.

* Prepare yourself, your family and friends practically and psychologically for your regime. You will need all the support you can get.

* It is worth taking some time off work to do it if you can. You will return as refreshed as if you had been

away on holiday and you can invest the money you would have spent otherwise on pampering yourself on massages, oils, etc. Alternatively, identify a suitable weekend when you could kick-start your regime with a fruit fast.

* Retreat from the social limelight for a while – you don't need to be tempted or to be made to feel indulgent or silly about what you are undertaking.

* If you can, persuade other people to do it with you. You will be able to cheer each other on when things are going well and commiserate when progress seems slow.

* Forward planning is essential if the regime is going to be a success. Make a list of the things that you need and have everything ready before you start. If you run out of fruit or feel uninspired by your salad materials, your resolve is much more likely to weaken.

* Weigh and measure yourself (hips, thighs, above knees, upper arms, etc) before you start and repeat at monthly intervals. You may experience a fairly dramatic weight loss initially as excess fluid is drained from your body. This should stabilise once you return to more normal eating patterns.

* Record your feelings and any physical changes in a diary or notebook. This is also a good way of monitoring your reactions to food and finding out your natural affinities and intolerances.

* Eat lightly on the day before you start.

Fruit Fast: Days 1–3

To call this a fast is a bit of a misnomer. Nevertheless, feeding your body nothing but fruit will stimulate all the benefits of fasting, namely the rest and recuperation of your liver, kidneys and digestive system plus the burn-up of toxic material, while keeping your metabolism ticking over.

The following fruits are recommended: apples, apricots, bananas, bilberries, blackberries, blackcurrants, blueberries, cherries, cranberries, dates, figs, grapes, greengages, guavas, kiwis, kumquats, lemons and limes (for juice), loganberries, lychees, mangoes, cantaloupe and watermelons, nectarines, papayas, passion fruit, peaches, pears, persimmons, pineapples, pomegranates, raspberries, satsumas, sharon fruit, star fruit, strawberries, tangerines.

Note: Do not feel you have to go out of your way to obtain the more exotic fruits. The list is intended to cater to a range of tastes and to include fruits that are available all the year round.

* Eat your fill of fresh uncooked fruit roughly every two hours or spread over five sittings. Abandon your normal meal-time routines for the moment and consume your pile of fruit in a comfortable chair, say, while you read the paper or watch the television. Sitting down to a laid table will only remind you of what you are missing.

* It is important to keep your consumption up to a certain level as the fruit has an active role in cleansing the system.

* Chew every mouthful thoroughly.

* If you don't find it too boring, stick to one type of

fruit per sitting to allow the beneficial properties of each fruit to work on your system.

* Eat melon on its own or leave a gap of twenty minutes before trying another type of fruit.

* Bananas stave off hunger pangs like no other fruit because they are full of starch, but they will slow down elimination. They should be eaten in moderation and only when ripe (go for the ones with tell-tale brown spots on the skin).

* Limit your consumption of dried fruits (unsulphured) and eat only after soaking them overnight in spring water. Drinking the water in which they have soaked is a good remedy for constipation.

* Avoid oranges and grapefruits at this stage, as they can be tough on your already overworked liver. Some people may find the enzyme bromelin in pineapple can have a slightly caustic effect in the mouth too.

* Stop eating any fruit you have a reaction to.

Liquids

* Start the day with a glass of cold or hot water spiked with a squeeze of fresh lemon to flush out the kidneys and cleanse the palate.

* Keep up your daily quota of water (if you are drinking mineral water go for still rather than carbonated, which is slightly acidic) to replace the liquid you will

almost certainly be losing through increased urination.

* Do not drink with food at this stage as it dilutes the digestive juices. Try to leave half an hour before and after eating.

* Replace coffee and tea with herbal drinks – up to three cups a day. Look out for early morning and bedtime varieties. Lemon verbena and lime blossom are refreshing wake-up teas. Dandelion is an excellent diuretic because it also tops up your potassium levels, but nettle and solidago tea are also recommended. Peppermint, fennel and camomile aid digestion.

* You can drink unsweetened fruit juice diluted with mineral water. Undiluted fruit juices are too acid for the stomach. They will also send your blood sugar levels reeling. Ideally, make your own with an automatic juicer (see my *Quick Guide to Juicing* published by Boxtree).

Comforts

* Have a stash of precooked brown rice in the fridge. You can then warm yourself up a bowl if you are beset by cravings and hunger pangs. This will not undermine your regime. Brown rice is an excellent detoxifying food as it is easily digested and readily absorbs the toxins released in the gut. You can use oatcakes for a similar purpose. Here is a method of cooking brown rice which ensures that you end up with plump, fluffy grains. Measure out two cups of

rice and wash thoroughly under running water. Put the rice in a pan with five cups of weak additive-free vegetable stock and a crushed clove of garlic. Bring to the boil. Cover the pan and leave to cook for the recommended time *undisturbed*. Remove from heat and leave to stand.

* Make up a mixture of raw sesame, pumpkin and sunflower seeds and eat a handful as a snack. Nutritionally speaking, these seeds are small gems, packed with protein, vitamins and minerals and the essential fatty acids which are indispensable for healthy skin. Store them in an air-tight jar to keep fresh. Never eat them if you suspect they might be rancid.

Other Options

If you don't feel you can manage on fruit alone for more than a day, then you can kick-start the regime with a twenty-four-hour fruit fast, before moving on to the next phase. Apples and pears are very cleansing and most effective for a single-fruit fast. Track down as many different types as possible for variety and eat as much of the fruit as possible.

Supplements

See Useful Addresses for suppliers.

* Take a full-spectrum multivitamin and mineral supplement for about six weeks to top up essential nutrients. This will also put right any long-term

deficiencies and provide additional support for the detox.

* A teaspoon of vitamin C powder mixed with a splash of diluted pure fruit juice and washed down with a glass of mineral water may help to relieve any headaches which arise during the early stages of the detox.

* Kelp is another useful cellulite-busting supplement. Like all seaweeds, it is high in iodine, which regulates the thyroid gland. This is responsible for controlling the body's metabolism – the rate at which it burns fat.

* Alfalfa is rich in micronutrients – the substances that the body requires in minute doses to survive – as well as certain enzymes necessary for digestion. Any supplement which limits the toxic build-up caused by partially digested food is relevant to cellulite. Alfalfa also contains the enzyme lipase, which is thought to be reduced in cellulite sufferers.

* The leaves of the ginkgo biloba tree are highly antioxidant and their bioflavonoid content helps to protect capillary walls. Ginkgo biloba extract, available in tablet form, helps to boost circulation. It is also currently being investigated for use in anti-cellulite creams.

* Silica is important for building connective tissue and improving the production of collagen and keratin, which provide the skin's underpinnings and top layer. Refined grains and vegetables grown in depleted soil contain reduced levels of silica, which the cellulite beater might wish to supplement.

Be Prepared

* Be prepared for side-effects – these may last for anything up to a week. They are likely to include a 'furry' tongue, increased urination, headaches, mood swings, diarrhoea and/or constipation, mouth ulcers, even the onset of a cold or flu. These are nevertheless positive signs and show that the toxins are on the move.

* 'Fasting headaches' occur as the toxins released by the liver into the bloodstream pass through the delicate capillaries of the brain. Take a draught of vitamin C (see Supplements above), drink additional mineral water, increase fruit consumption or go for a gentle walk to relieve these. You can also try gently pressing the acupressure point in the sensitive fleshy region between your thumb and index finger for up to a minute on each hand.

* Put on an extra layer or curl up with a hot water bottle if you are feeling chilly. Also consider grating some fresh ginger in a glass of hot lemon water or a herbal tea to warm the system. Spice fanatics might enjoy ginger tea.

* Have an afternoon nap if you can and feel like it. Go to bed as early as possible. Don't be surprised if you wake up earlier than usual.

* Exercise will speed up the removal of toxins through perspiration, exhalation and improved circulation of the blood and lymphatic system. However, you probably will not have the energy to do much during the first week.

Fruit and Vegetable Fast: Days 7–10

The next phase introduces raw and some cooked vegetables into the regime, as well as additional carbohydrates. You should not feel deprived or hungry on this diet so do not stint on quantity.

Recommended vegetables include: asparagus, avocados, beans, beetroot, broccoli, Brussels sprouts, cabbage (red, white or green), carrots, cauliflower, celery, chicory, courgettes, cress, cucumber, endive, fennel, garlic, kale, leeks, lettuces, mangetout, marrow, onions (all types), parsnips, peas, peppers, pumpkin, radishes, salad leaves of all kinds (especially red leaves), squashes, swede, turnip, watercress.

* Start the day with lemon water.

* Eat as much fruit as you like for breakfast and as a mid-morning or mid-afternoon snack.

* Drink water or herb teas freely, away from meals.

* Try hot vegetable bouillon (available in powder form from all good health shops) and vegetable juices (carrot, beetroot, V8), which can also be lightly warmed in cooler weather.

* Make yourself a huge raw vegetable salad for lunch and supper – as much as you can eat. You can serve it with a dressing (cold-pressed sunflower/safflower or extra virgin olive oil, fresh lemon juice or cider vinegar, parsley or other fresh herbs and garlic). Alternatively, liquidise chopped raw vegetables and add olive oil and a splash of lemon juice to create a raw vegetable soup.

* Sprinkle sesame, pumpkin and sunflower seeds, whole or ground, liberally on to your salads.

* Vegetable soups, ie fresh vegetables cooked in additive-free vegetable stock, make a comforting accompaniment to a big salad.

* Or try potatoes baked or steamed in their skins and garnished with olive oil and chopped parsley, chives or nori flakes (see below).

* Use brown rice as a base for a very satisfying raw vegetable salad.

* Chop avocados into your salads or use them to make dressings or a dip for crudités.

* Sprouted seeds, grains and beans (including mung beans, alfalfa, sunflower seeds, wholewheat and lentils) are an almost ideal source of nutrition and will complement any salad. You can buy them ready-sprouted or grow them yourself in a special sprouting container or using a jam jar covered with a piece of muslin.

* Sea vegetables (eg kelp, nori, wakami – available from oriental and health food shops) are packed with iodine which can help to speed up your metabolism and maintain a steady rate of detoxification. They are also a remarkable source of vitamins and minerals and contain 25 percent more protein than milk. Alginic acid in seaweed is believed to bind with toxins and remove them from the system. Sprinkle nori flakes on soups and use as an alternative to chives in

cottage cheese. You can also wrap fish in nori sheets
before baking.

Please Note

* Incorporate all the things you like and be as
  imaginative as you can with colours and textures –
  there is no reason for your diet to be boring.

* Plan your meals in advance and shop specifically for
  them so that you always have something to look
  forward to. Rifle through recipe books for inspiration.

A Final Word

Different diets suit different people and huge quantities of raw
foods, with precious little to adulterate them, are not everybody's ideal. If you are in this category, you would do better to
skip the fruit and vegetable fasts altogether and go straight on to
the Healthy Eating Plan below. If, on the other hand, you are
unaccustomed to a diet so high in raw foods, but do not think
it would disagree with your system, give it a try. You are unlikely
to regret it.

A Gentler Approach

If you feel, for whatever reason, that you cannot incorporate the
fruit and vegetable fasts into your working or domestic life, you
can start your anti-cellulite diet here. The results will not be as
quick if you miss out the detoxification stage, but with all the
toxifying elements excluded, and the emphasis placed heavily

on nourishing and cleansing with pure, natural foods, the eating plan which follows will nevertheless set you on the right course.

For those who have completed the fruit and/or vegetable fasts, this phase is a logical progression from the first part of the anti-cellulite diet and adds a variety of wholegrains, pulses, fish, meat, eggs and nuts to the raw fruit and vegetable core.

HEALTHY EATING PLAN

* Eat regularly.

* Whatever you do, don't skip breakfast. It will only leave you vulnerable to cravings later on in the morning.

* Continue with a fruit breakfast if you are happy on it. Fruit smoothies, made in a blender using whatever combination of fruits you fancy, are a pleasant variation. Adding a banana gives smoothies a bit more substance.

* Breakfast alternatives include:
  – unsweetened wholegrain muesli soaked overnight in fruit juice and eaten with live low-fat yoghurt
  – 10oz live yoghurt topped with a sliced banana and a generous handful of seeds
  – porridge served with a little honey, chopped dates or a banana and a sprinkling of cinnamon
  – a slice of toast spread with mashed banana and a teaspoon of tahini.

* Make a large salad of raw vegetables the centrepiece of one meal a day and incorporate a salad or steamed vegetables into the other one.

* As an alternative, stir-fry your vegetables in a small amount of cold-pressed sesame oil or experiment with different ways of baking them. Using a non-stick frying pan will require you to use less oil.

* Incorporate unlimited quantities of garlic and fresh herbs.

You can now reintroduce the following foods:

* Wholegrains. Oats, rye, barley (best in soups), buckwheat (including spaghetti), millet and polenta, in addition to the staple brown rice.

* Raw, unsalted nuts. Cashews, brazils, almonds, chestnuts, hazelnuts, walnuts, pecans and pine kernels. Avoid peanuts and coconut.

* Pulses. Lentils, split peas, chick peas, haricot, borlotti, flageolet and kidney beans, to name a few. They can be incorporated into hot soups, curries, casseroles and served cold in hummus, salads, etc. Eat with rice or grains. These are useful slow-releasing carbohydrates which can keep you satisfied for hours. To minimise flatulence, soak pulses overnight then discard water. Cook with a clove of garlic.

* Fish. White (cod, haddock, hake, coley), oily (herring, mackerel, salmon, tuna, sardine, anchovy) and shellfish. Eat three or four times per week.

* Meat. Restrict consumption to once a week. Try to track down a butcher who supplies free-range, additive-free organic meat and choose lamb, game or

poultry. Trim off excess fat and buy 'extra-lean' where possible. Remove skin from poultry before eating. Grill, bake or stew.

* Free-range eggs. No more than three per week.

* Investigate tofu for use in stir-fries and dips. Needs marinating to acquire any flavour.

* Restrict wheat consumption to once a day – wholewheat bread and flour products, cracked wheat (or bulgar), couscous. Try the following breads and biscuits as alternatives to those made with wheat: 100 percent rye bread, pumpernickel bread, rye biscuits (Finn Crisp high fibre are nice and chunky with good flavour), Scottish oatcakes, whole-grain pittas and chapattis, whole-corn tortillas, and rice cakes.

* Keep your intake of dairy products down to a minimum. If you do eat cheese, try to make sure it's soft and low fat (eg ricotta or cottage cheese) and use it as a garnish rather than a centrepiece. Sheep and goats' cheeses are preferable to those made with cows' milk. Cream is for feast days only. Use an unhydrogenated margarine like Vitaquell (available from health food shops) for spreading, and a small quantity of cold-pressed extra virgin olive oil or unrefined sesame oil for cooking.

'SAFE' SNACKS

Provided you are snacking on the right kind of foods, there is nothing wrong with eating between meals to give your blood sugar levels a boost when they are starting to flag. Here are some ideas:

* Fresh fruit, eaten as it comes or whizzed up into a cool frappé or a smoothie

* Raw vegetables: carrots, celery, cucumber, peppers, radishes

* Sunflower and pumpkin seeds

* Natural yoghurt with a sprinkling of seeds

* Oatcakes, rice cakes, rye biscuits

* Toast with banana and/or tahini

* Fresh nuts, in moderation

* Small bowl of muesli

FOOD COMBINING

This system, evolved in the 1920s by Dr William Hay, is relevant to anyone who suffers from poor elimination or indigestion. Dr Hay believed that food groups with different digestive properties should not be mixed in one meal because they tend to result in incomplete digestion. Carbohydrate-rich foods (potatoes, rice, pasta, bread or other grains) are broken down in an alkaline environment, while the presence of protein (meat, fish, eggs, cheese, or milk) stimulates acid secretion. If you combine them together, your body gets involved in a battle to treat each of the intermingled foodstuffs in the appropriate way, resulting in a lot of poorly digested and assimilated food.

AVOID OR SEVERELY RESTRICT

* Cigarettes and tobacco

* Spirits

* Fried foods

* Smoked foods (these are often highly salted and coloured as well)

* Beef and pork

* Preserved/prepared meats (bacon, sausages, salami, pâté, etc)

* Processed and junk food

* Salted snacks, ie crisps, nuts, etc

* Refined carbohydrates (pies, pastries, biscuits, cakes, white bread, white rice)

* Sugars

* Carbonated drinks and squashes

* Chocolate, confectionery and ice-cream

Special cases

* If, after two weeks of total abstinence, you are really desperate for a shot of caffeine, you can allow yourself one cup daily of freshly ground coffee from beans kept in the freezer, or one–two cups of tea.

* A glass of red wine with your evening meal won't hurt. It may even act as a digestive. Do not get into

the habit of drinking every day, though, and always try to consume alcohol *with* food. It is worth finding a palatable organic wine to minimise the toxic element.

MEAL PLANNING

Start by building up a repertoire of salads, which you can make the main focus of a meal or have in a supporting role. These salads will inevitably change from one season to the next according to the produce that is available. Then work on your soups. They are one of the best ways of preserving the goodness of cooked vegetables and can provide the basis for a light meal or an introduction to a more substantial one. Don't forget that chilled soups are very refreshing in summer.

Try out different ways of preparing vegetables to serve with your fish or meat. Alternatively, you may prefer to eat a clutch of vegetables together with some pulses and grains. Proteins will be playing a modest role in your diet, but don't neglect them. Experiment with new cooking methods and ingredients to find out how you can maximise the flavour as well as the nutritional value. Try to make the savoury element of your meal so satisfying that you don't even think about pudding.

The following suggestions should help to get you started.

Soups

Raw tomato soup
Iced avocado soup
Cold spinach, lentil and yoghurt soup
Hot or cold beetroot soup
Harvest/winter vegetable soup
Leek and potato soup
Curried parsnip soup
Shrimp and potato soup
Chicken mulligatawny soup

Starters and salads

Crudités and guacamole/cottage cheese

Roasted/grilled peppers in vinaigrette

Steamed corn on the cob

Tomato, goats' cheese and basil salad

Spinach or curly endive salad garnished with chopped hard-
boiled eggs and sesame seeds

Main courses/light meals

Baked potato with cottage cheese and nori flakes with a salad of red
cabbage, celeriac, carrot and mung bean sprouts

Hummus and pittas served with radicchio and chicory salad

Gazpacho followed by pasta salad incorporating spring vegetables
and pine nuts

Lentil soup and a brown rice salad made with carrot, celery, pepper
and tomato

Minestrone soup, served with radicchio and Chinese leaf salad and
rye toast spread with olive paste

Stir-fry of buckwheat spaghetti, broccoli and mushrooms garnished
with sesame seeds with a Chinese leaf and watercress salad

Feta salad with lettuce, tomatoes, peppers, cucumber and alfalfa
sprouts served with wholemeal pittas

Salade niçoise made with steamed new potatoes and fresh grilled
tuna

Grilled chicken breast brushed with pesto with seasonal steamed
vegetables

Lamb or vegetarian couscous served with avocado and red leaf
salad

Grilled salmon steaks with a warm salad of lightly steamed broccoli and courgettes

Baked white fish in yoghurt marinade served with braised fennel
and brown rice

Grilled lamb chops served with roasted ratatouille and buckwheat
pilaff

Postscript

There's room in any regime for feast days, so enjoy them rather than agonise over them. When your body is well nourished and spring-cleaned, it will be much better able to cope anyway. Follow your instinct. If you feel you are suffering from toxic overload, give your system a rest. Have a day eating just fruit or raw vegetables and you'll soon bounce back.

—— 5 ——
Treatment and Therapies

In addition to the efforts you can make with your diet, your exercise plan and your bathing routines, there is a whole world of products out there boasting about their cellulite-reducing powers, which you may be tempted to buy, or at least would like to know a little more about.

It has to be said that anti-cellulite creams, lotions, gels and oils are very unlikely to have any more than a light toning or firming effect, if they are not backed up by dietary changes and increased physical activity.

Massage is usually recommended once the cream has been applied, as it encourages the ingredients to penetrate the lower levels of the skin. Massage also stimulates the circulation beneath the skin, bringing warmth to the area. 'Thermogenic' creams contain ingredients which do the warming for you. In the absence of skin brushing, exfoliating scrubs take over the job of removing the dead skin cells and cleansing the pores. This enhances the skin's capacity to absorb the active ingredients.

The Plant World

So what do these products contain that could conceivably have an effect on cellulite? Thanks to the 'greening' of toiletries which has taken place over the last five or six years, the plant kingdom has been ransacked. The therapeutic properties of berries, beans, bark, roots, leaves and any other part of a plant you care to mention are being tested for their effectiveness in treating the problems of cellulite. Manufacturers are also jumping on the aromatherapy bandwagon and including essential oils in the cocktail.

Broadly speaking, the plant extracts and essential oils favoured for combating cellulite contain ingredients capable of a range of actions. They include strengthening the blood vessels and boosting circulation, draining the waterlogged tissue, reducing inflammation, soothing nerves and muscles, and tightening and softening the skin. The extent of the action depends on how deep the substance is able to penetrate.

AROMATHERAPY

Aromatherapy uses our sense of smell to treat a range of disorders, or simply to enhance our well-being. The essential oils, or aromatic essences, are known to permeate the system by two different paths. Smell is the quickest route to the brain, which may explain why certain aromas have the capacity to alter our moods, easing anxieties and even lifting depression. Essential oils also filter into the bloodstream, where they can work on the blood and the vessels of the circulatory system. Like vitamins, they act therapeutically on the organs of the body with which they have an affinity.

Aromatherapy has many applications in the anti-cellulite regime. Not only can you advance the cause with aromatic baths and aromatherapy massages, you can also inhale the therapeutic aromas as you go about the house, by burning the oils in a special device and even putting a drop on to light bulbs. A couple of words of warning. It is important to obtain your essential oils from a reliable source, since their effectiveness rests on the quality of the raw materials and the extraction methods used. Essential oils are costly because so little is extracted from each plant, but they are powerful, so a little goes a long way.

Different oils possess different qualities and there are a number of aromatic essences specifically recommended for the treatment of cellulite. These include basil, cedarwood, celery, cypress, fennel, grapefruit, juniper, lemon, oregano, patchouli, rosemary, sage and thyme. The following blends will work on reducing fluid retention, revving up circulation and eliminating toxins. They will also help to relieve any tenderness in the tissue and improve the skin tone. Always use the exact number of drops suggested and keep oils tightly sealed in dark glass bottles away from direct heat.

Mix your own
Essential oils work in the bath by osmosis, as well as aromatically (don't forget to keep the bathroom door closed so that the precious aromas do not escape). It is worth having a number of blends to hand so you can rotate them, as the body ceases to respond as well once it gets used to a particular mixture. Also, you will find some combinations more appealing than others. Soak in your bath for at least ten minutes – ideally for fifteen or twenty.

Anti-cellulite baths
   A   *8 drops thyme + 4 drops lemon*
   B   *8 drops sage + 4 drops patchouli*
   C   *6 drops rosemary + 6 drops juniper*
   D   *6 drops oregano + 6 drops lemon*

Follow your bath with a massage with one of these **anti-cellulite massage oils**.

To 4fl oz grapeseed oil and 1tsp wheat germ oil add:
   A   *10 drops juniper + 5 drops mandarin + 5 drops fennel*
   B   *8 drops grapefruit + 6 drops fennel + 6 drops lemon*

You can also help to activate affected areas by massaging in this home-made **anti-cellulite scrub**.

> *2tbsp finely ground adzuki beans or lentils*
> *1 level tbsp coarsely ground oatmeal*
> *1tbsp grapeseed oil*
> *2 tbsp witch hazel*
> *6 drops juniper or cypress*

Blend ingredients to form a thick paste. Using the palms of your hands, firmly massage across your thighs, hips and buttocks. Rub the surface of the skin with circular movements, massaging the entire area for at least three minutes before showering off with alternate blasts of cool and icy water.

If you wish to sample a professional aromatherapy massage, follow up a personal recommendation or contact the International Federation of Aromatherapists for a list of registered practitioners (see Useful Addresses). Your aromatherapist will take a full case history before selecting the appropriate oils to deal with your particular cellulite symptoms.

SEAWEED AND SEA WATER

We have already touched on the benefits of seaweeds, beloved by orientals and north Europeans, in our food. What you fail to take in by mouth, you can now absorb through the skin in the form of seaweed soaps, bath products, body creams and body wraps. It appears that seaweed has a lot to offer us. In 1897 René Quinton, a French doctor, observed the similarity between sea water and human plasma: 'In the internal environment of our body, and only there, do we find the same mineral make-up as that of sea water.'

Seaweeds are like a concentrate of sea water, easily usable by man and packed with all the minerals, vitamins, amino acids and trace elements required to nourish the skin. A gallon of seaweed, carefully preserved and processed, contains the same quantity of nutrients as 10,000 gallons of sea water. Its pureness (when it has not been grown in polluted waters) arises from the fact that it is derived from a single substance – the sea – which has a pretty constant composition and rarely has any deficiencies. You may be wondering how plants grown in soil can possibly compete?

The interest that seaweed holds for the cellulite sufferer concerns its ability to stimulate the circulation and the flow of oxygen to the skin's deepest layer. This activates the exchange of substances, speeding up the elimination of toxins and increasing the flow of nutrients to rebalance and remineralise the skin. There are other benefits too. The iodine element in seaweed works on the thyroid gland to speed up the body's metabolism and burn up both toxins and unwanted fat. High levels of potassium rid the system of excess water.

It has been scientifically proven using radioactive tracers that the constituent elements of sea water do penetrate the subcutaneous layer of the skin. Thalassotherapy, a term coined by a French doctor in 1869 to describe the therapeutic use of seaweed and seawater, is readily available on the Continent and increasingly in the UK.

ALL SYSTEMS GO
Practically every anti-cellulite product on the market contains some kind of diuretic, a substance which increases the flow of urine and therefore reduces the amount of fluid in the body. Caffeine, ivy, horsetail, butcher's broom, hawkweed, fennel, juniper and patchouli are all used for this purpose. Arguably, this is where the effectiveness of a lot of the products lies. If you remove the puffiness associated with cellulite which is caused by fluid retention, you will inevitably improve the look and feel of the skin.

Plant extracts and oils used to tone and stimulate the circulatory system are also an important ingredient in anti-cellulite preparations. Some of the popular raw materials with these properties include ivy, hawkweed, cypress, butcher's broom, rosemary, marjoram, geranium, horse chestnut and caffeine. They improve the blood flow by widening the arteries. In addition, ivy, hawkweed, butcher's broom and ginkgo biloba extract all contain vitamins called bioflavonoids which strengthen weak blood vessels as well (a common problem among cellulite sufferers).

Astringents are an important feel-good factor in these creams. They stimulate the cell walls to contract, thereby condensing the tissue and making it firmer. Horsetail, hawkweed and horse chestnut feature in the lists of ingredients, along with rosemary, sandalwood and geranium. Like the diuretics, they produce instant, if short-lived, improvements. Other skin beautifiers include the softening agent aloe vera, wheatgerm and vitamin E to nourish and protect the skin and geranium and patchouli for their toning properties. Hazelnut oil and tea seed oil are chosen for their enriching and lubricating properties.

Caffeine and its derivatives are a staple ingredient in anti-cellulite products. When applied to the skin, caffeine is believed to be able to penetrate deep enough to stimulate the combustion of the fat cells in areas like the thighs and buttocks. Available from six different plant species, including the coffee tree, the cacao tree, the tea tree and the Amazonian guarana, it is used in apparently harmless concentrations of between 1 and 2 percent. Judging by French research which showed no change in caffeine levels in blood before and after the use of the cellulite cream, systemic absorption does not seem to be a risk.

One of the most significant developments in the 'cosmaceutical' laboratories over the past few years has been the creation of 'microparticles', 'microspheres', 'nanospheres', and other vehicles to convey the active ingredients to affected areas. This technical refinement ensures that the active ingredients are not released until they reach the real trouble spots. In addition, these vehicles have a built-in delaying factor, which allows them to prolong the release over a twenty-four-hour period. Trials using these new products show an improvement in skin tissue after between fifteen days' and thirty days' use, continuing for up to three months.

AMINOPHYLLINE

The latest arrival on the anti-cellulite shelf, billed as a 'wonder-drug' capable of shrinking thighs without even the effort of massage, is aminophylline. The drug has long been used in low concentrations to treat asthma, but Frank Greenaway, an endocrinologist at UCLA, and George Bray, Professor of Medicine at Louisiana State University, first became interested in its fat-burning potential in 1978.

It appears that aminophylline, along with its close relative theophylline, belongs to the same group of drugs as caffeine. Like caffeine, it is capable of interfering with the normal hormonal action to preserve the fat cells on the thighs at all costs, by blocking the relevant messages to the cells. This allows the cells to release their fat stores more easily and, according to studies carried out over the last decade, to slim the thighs of 80 percent of the women who use it.

The jury is still out on these products, recently launched on both sides of the Atlantic. The diuretic effect of aminophylline, when taken internally, suggests that the reduction in thigh girth is due to fluid loss. And there are a number of questions which still need to be asked. Is it advisable to apply a preparation containing a drug to a part of the body with such powers of absorption as the skin?

Dr Richard James describes aminophylline as 'not inordinately toxic' and a 2 percent concentration applied locally does not seem to him to be inherently risky. Nor does he view the prospect of a flood of fatty acids suddenly entering the bloodstream as a potential health hazard. However, without an associated exercise programme offering the body the possibility of burning up the liberated fatty acids, it is not inconceivable that they might end up being laid down in the fatty tissue at a later date.

Aminophylline is also administered in a technique called mesotherapy, which has recently been introduced into this country. Mesotherapy is a conventional medical technique, widely used in France and Belgium, to treat a range of conditions including arthritis and back pain, as well as cellulite. The word mesotherapy means therapy at the site of the disorder. Treatment involves injecting two teaspoons of a cocktail of medicines, prescribed by a doctor individually for each patient, using a tiny needle. A device resembling a small air gun forces the droplets 2–3mm under the skin to where the cellulite is.

The concentration of aminophylline injected represents between a twentieth and a fiftieth of the standard adult oral dose. Dr Elisabeth Dancey, who discovered mesotherapy while practising as a GP in Belgium and now practices it in London, admits that the aminophylline can produce a reaction in sensitive people in the form of a localised rash. Other elements in the cocktail include something to boost the flow of blood and lymph, an enzyme to dissolve the fibrous capsule which envelops the fat cells, and a small amount of local anaesthetic, which helps to ensure that the medicine remains in the tissue rather than entering the bloodstream.

The combination of drugs is designed to reverse the causes of the cellulite. Ninety percent of women apparently benefit from the treatment, achieving a lasting reduction of 1–2cm over ten to fifteen sessions; but at a considerable cost. Patients are also encouraged to make changes in their diet, with a total ban on junk food, fried food, artificial sweeteners, fizzy drinks, chocolate, sweets, cakes, biscuits and ice-cream. Regular exercise is also recommended.

CELLULOLIPOLYSIS

This is another treatment popular in France which is now available in this country. It is meant to be particularly effective in treating stubborn deposits. After a fitness check with a qualified doctor and a urine analysis, to check sodium and potassium levels in the body, your vital statistics are fed into a machine, which then prescribes the necessary treatment. Sodium and/or potassium supplements are suggested where necessary and all patients are encouraged to drink two litres of water daily and to follow a low-fat diet.

During the treatment, up to eight electrodes (needles no thicker than a hair) are placed under the skin over the cellulite deposits on outer thighs and inner knees. The tissue is then subjected to a high speed vibration, which is intended to break down the hardened nodules. Supposedly, results are noticeable after three weeks of a course of six or eight treatments and continue for up to six weeks after the treatment ends. Light bruising is not uncommon. You might need to take out a small mortgage to pay for this. Some women have also found cellulolipolysis extremely painful, 'like childbirth' claimed one tester, with little visible difference at the end of the treatments.

IONITHERMIE

Some of the treatments available in a salon setting combine technology with natural ingredients. Ionithermie involves applying a thermal clay mask (containing ivy, bile (extracted from cows' innards!), seaweed extracts, vitamins, amino acids and azulen) to affected areas to draw out toxins while administering two types of 'therapeutic' electric current – galvanic and faradic. The idea is that the galvanic current propels the active ingredients deep into the skin to break down fat, fluid and toxins and stimulate the blood and lymphatic systems to eliminate wastes. In addition the faradic current, used by medical physiotherapists to help restore weak and injured tissue, stimulates muscles electrically.

LYMPHATIC DRAINAGE

If you are going to invest in some professional treatment, it is worth considering a proper lymphatic drainage massage. In an ideal world, say some healthcare experts, we would all have one a week for the rest of our lives. Carried out by a trained professional, it can have a dramatic effect, improving the exchanges between cells and interstitial fluid and speeding up removal of cellular wastes.

Tension in the body will reduce the effectiveness of lymphatic drainage massage, which is why the technique is rarely used in isolation. Barbara Tait, a therapist at the London College of Massage, combines lymphatic drainage with a relaxing general massage, as well as working on knotted muscles. This creates an uninterrupted circuit round which the blood and lymph can flow. She explains, 'Chronic muscle tension acts like a dam: blood doesn't want to go in and toxins don't want to leave.'

When the system becomes sluggish and ineffective the lymph vessels are usually congested. The pumping and gentle circular movements of lymphatic drainage massage can clear the blockages and gently push the lymph in the direction of the lymph nodes, where the impurities are filtered out, before returning via the lymph ducts to the blood stream. It is also possible to improve lymphatic drainage using mechanical massage techniques available in some health and beauty clinics.

OTHER THERAPIES

There are other therapies which may be helpful in addressing specific physiological problems such as poor lymphatic drainage, while bringing additional benefits. **Shiatsu**, or Japanese 'finger pressure' therapy, stimulates the body's vital energy flow by the same principles as acupuncture. Fingers and thumbs, elbows and sometimes even knees and feet are used to apply pressure to the energy lines known as meridians. This boosts the circulation and the flow of lymphatic fluid, releasing toxins and tension from muscles. Shiatsu also strengthens the nervous system and restores calm to the body.

Postural imbalances may be helped by the **Alexander technique** or **Rolfing**, both of which attempt to release the muscles from habitual or damaging positioning, the latter by connective tissue manipulation. **Osteopathy** will address any structural difficulties, particularly problems relating to the spine. This is done primarily through manipulation of the joints in order to restore them to their normal positions and mobility, thereby relieving abnormal tension in muscles and ligaments.

AND FINALLY ...

A number of these treatments and therapies involve handing the responsibility over to other people to deal with your cellulite. Professional assistance can, of course, be valuable and involving an objective third party may act as an incentive for some. However, having it all done for you does not help you to address the real causes and to evolve a way of reducing cellulite now and in the future. Cellulite can always return, if you have a predisposition to it. So, be prepared and be on your guard. Good luck!

Glossary

Bioflavonoid – A nutrient that works with vitamin C to maintain blood vessels, especially the small capillaries, and acts as an anti-inflammatory agent.

Collagen – Chief component and strengthening element in fibrous connective tissue. Requires vitamin C for its formation.

Diuretic – Any substance that increases the flow of urine from the body.

Endocrine system – A collection of glands which secrete hormones into the bloodstream.

Enzyme – A substance produced by living cells which acts as a catalyst in certain chemical processes within the body.

Free radicals – Highly reactive molecules produced as a natural by-product of body chemistry which attack, infiltrate and damage vital cell structures.

Interstitial – Occurring in the spaces between the cells.

Lymphatic system – An extensive network of capillary vessels that transports the interstitial fluid of the body as lymph to the venous blood circulation.

Microcirculation – The circulation of blood or lymph in the finest blood vessels or capillaries of the circulatory and lymphatic systems.

Plasma – The liquid part of blood or lymph.

Useful Addresses

Bodytreats International Ltd
15 Approach Road
London SW20 8BA
Tel: 0181-543 5633
Essential oils and anti-cellulite blends by mail order.

The Cellulite Clinic
London College of Massage
5–6 Newman Passage
London W1 3PF
Tel: 0171-637 7125
Lymphatic drainage massage and nutritional advice.

General Council and Register of Osteopaths
56 London Road
Reading
Berkshire RG1 9SQ
Tel: 01734 576585
Contact for a list of registered osteopaths.

International Federation of Aromatherapists
4 Eastmearn Road
West Dulwich
London SE21 8HA
Tel: 01455 637987
Contact for a list of registered aromatherapists.

Larkhall Green Farm
225 Putney Bridge Road
London SW15 2PY
Tel: 0181-874 1130
Body brushes and nutritional supplements by mail order.

Micheline Arcier
7 William Street
London SW1X 9HL
Tel: 0171-235 3545
Essential oils and anti-cellulite blends by mail order.

Neal's Yard Remedies
5 Golden Cross
Cornmarket Street
Oxford OX1 3EU
Tel: 01865 245436
Essential oils and anti-cellulite blends by mail order.

The Nutri Centre
7 Park Crescent
London W1N 3HE
Tel: 0171-436 5122
Nutritional supplements by mail order.

PT Leisure Ltd
New Rock House
Dymock
Gloucestershire GL18 2BB
Tel: 01531 890888
Rebounders.

Shirley Price Aromatherapy
Wesley House
Stockwell Road
Hinckley
Leicestershire LE10 1RD
Tel: 01455 615466
Essential oils and anti-cellulite blends by mail order.

Society of Teachers of the Alexander Technique
20 London House
266 Fulham Road
London SW10 9EL
Tel: 0171-351 0828
Send an A5 SAE for a list of recognised teachers in the UK.

The Soil Association
86 Colston Street
Bristol BS1 5BB
Tel: 0117 929 0661
Contact for a list of local suppliers of organic produce.

Tisserand Aromatherapy Supplies
The Knoll Business Centre
Old Shoreham Road
Hove
East Sussex BN3 7GS
Tel: 01273 412139
Essential oils and anti-cellulite blends by mail order.

Index

HOW TO ORDER YOUR BOXTREE BOOKS BY LIZ EARLE

❏ 0 7522 0558 7	Aromatherapy	£3.99
❏ 1 85283 544 3	Baby and Toddler Foods	£3.99
❏ 1 85283 543 5	Food Facts	£3.99
❏ 1 85283 546 X	Vegetarian Cookery	£3.99
❏ 0 7522 1619 8	Evening Primrose Oil	£3.99
❏ 0 7533 1614 7	Herbs for Health	£3.99
❏ 1 85283 984 8	Successful Slimming	£3.99
❏ 0 7522 0553 6	Vitamins and Minerals	£3.99
❏ 1 85283 979 1	Detox	£3.99
❏ 0 7522 1635 X	Hair Loss	£3.99
❏ 0 7522 0544 7	Youthful Skin	£3.99
❏ 0 7522 1680 5	Healthy Pregnancy	£3.99
❏ 0 7522 0548 X	Dry Skin and Eczema	£3.99
❏ 0 7522 1641 4	Cod Liver Oil	£3.99
❏ 0 7522 1626 0	Juicing	£3.99
❏ 0 7522 1631 7	Acne	£3.99
❏ 0 7522 1673 2	Food Combining	£3.99
❏ 0 7522 1690 2	Post-natal Health	£3.99
❏ 0 7522 1675 9	Food Allergies	£3.99
❏ 0 7522 1685 6	Healthy Menopause	£3.99
❏ 0 7522 1668 6	Beating PMS	£3.99
❏ 0 7522 1663 5	Antioxidants	£3.99
❏ 1 85283 518 4	Liz Earle's Ace Plan The New Guide to Super Vitamins A, C and E	£4.99
❏ 1 85283 554 0	Liz Earle's Ace Plan Weight-Loss for Life	£4.99
❏ 0 7522 0517 X	Liz Earle's New Bikini Diet	£4.99

All the books shown opposite are available at your local bookshop or can be ordered direct from the publisher. Just tick the titles you want and fill in the form below. Prices and availability subject to change without notice.

Boxtree Cash Sales,
PO Box 11, Falmouth, Cornwall TR10 9EN

Please send cheque or postal order for the value of the book(s), and add the following for postage and packing:

UK including BFPO – £1.00 for one book, plus 50p for the second book, and 30p for each additional book ordered up to a £3.00 maximum.
Overseas including Eire – £2.00 for the first book, plus £1.00 for the second book, and 50p for each additional book ordered.

OR
please debit this amount from my Access/VISA card (delete as appropriate)

Card number ☐☐☐☐☐☐☐☐☐☐☐☐☐☐☐☐

Amount £ ....

Expiry date on card ....

Signed ....

Name ....

Address ....

....

....